The
Skinny Rules

The
Skinny Rules

*Start to get skinny in just 24
hours with these 7 simple rules*

by

Edita Kaye

Important Please Read Carefully

The information, ideas, suggestions, and answers to questions in this book are not intended to substitute for the services of a physician. You should only undertake a fat loss, weight loss, or health modification program in conjunction with the services of a qualified health care professional. This book is intended as a reference guide only, not as a manual for self-treatment. If you suspect you have a medical problem or have questions, please talk to your own health care professional. All the information here is based on research available at the time of this printing.

Printed in the United States of America
October 2001

First Printing
ISBN   0-9635150-0-4

Other Books by Edita Kaye

The Skinny Pill
The Fountain of Youth
Bone Builders

Praise for Edita's *Skinny Solution* ™

I got my waist back. I'm tucking in my shirt and wearing a belt for the first time in years.
Nancy, Florida

I lost seven pounds in the first seven days!
Margaret, Washington

My husband lost over 30 pounds, lowered his cholesterol and blood pressure. You saved his life. Thank you.
Pam, Ohio

My daughter lost 25 pounds and her friends at school don't tease her anymore. Thank you for helping my little girl be happy, again.

Sheila & Dot, Minnesota

I actually wake up skinnier then when I go to bed. This is remarkable!

Sophie, Arkansas

We were always ashamed about our Mom. She was so fat. We didn't want her to come to parent's night at our school 'cause she was too fat to fit into the chairs. She got your book. She got skinny. Thank you.

Jennifer & Jody, Texas

Meet Edita

*America's Favorite Nutritionist
and the woman who's getting America
skinny again with great advice, laughter and
a prayer!!*

Edita is the author of the best selling, *The Skinny Pill* book and the creator of *The Skinny Pill™*, *Skinny Sleep™* and *Skinny Carbs™* Dietary Supplements.

She is also the author of *The Fountain of Youth* and *Bone Builders*, both published by Warner Books in New York.

She is the executive producer and host of the national PBS series, *The Fountain of Youth*.

Edita's books have been selected by the *Doubleday Book Club, the Literary Guild* and the *Christian Book Club*.

She has been featured in *Parade Magazine, USA Weekend, Ladies' Home Journal, Redbook, Woman's World,* and *First for Women.*

She has appeared on *QVC, HGTV, Fox National News*, and is a frequent guest on *Good Morning Texas*.

You Are Not Alone

This little book is part of the journey that is my life. My path has not always been smooth or even clear. I've been lost. I've been alone. Unloved. Abused. Broke. Scared. And I've been FAT.

But even during the worst moments…when everything was darkest…when I hated my own body…when I couldn't shut off the negative thoughts spinning in my brain…when even my soul felt bruised…at those very worst moments…a hand reached out to me…a voice whispered…and I knew I wasn't alone.

I'd like to share some of those moments with you and to reassure you that as you read this little book, you too, are not alone. I'm here. My Skinny counselors are here. My Skinny Rules are here. My whole Skinny Solution is here. It's simple. Just reach out.

1-888-7-SKINNY

www.skinny.com

A Special Thanks

I would like to offer a special thanks to all
those…

…who helped me with a hug when hugs
where in short supply.
…who gave me a smile when smiles were
hard to come by…
…who stood by me in good times, and most
importantly in the bad times…

God bless and keep you all.

Dedication

To everyone who has ever wished for simple rules to follow to get skinny fast, and stay skinny for life!

Table of Contents

Part Three: Make The Skinny Rules Part Of Your Life

Part One

Skinny Is Just A Day Away

"Why sometimes I've believed as many as six impossible things before breakfast."

Louis Carroll
Through the Looking Glass

It's never too late to be what you might have been.

George Eliot

My Own Skinny Story

I'm often asked what made me America's favorite nutritionist? What made me decide to dedicate my life to making America skinny? Healthy? Strong?

Those hundreds of thousands of you who read my book, *The Skinny Pill*, already know the story of how I found the exciting secret to the ultimate skinny solution.

But the real beginning happened several years before I created the formula for my skinny supplements. It happened years before I unlocked the secrets of skinny foods.

It happened when I was at the lowest point of my life. I haven't told this story to anyone before. But I would like to tell it to you now. I'd like to tell you the story of the day that changed my life forever. I hope it may change yours.

Even now, I can hardly believe what happened to me on that day which dawned in such darkness for me and ended with such blazing light.

It was just two weeks before my birthday. There I sat, on the floor of a motel room, surrounded by twenty-seven green garbage bags—stuffed to bursting with everything I owned. My life as I knew it, had ended.

I found myself abused. Broke. Homeless. Alone. I was in pain. I was old. I was scared—and oh, yes, as if all that weren't enough, I was FAT!

I felt so completely without hope. How was I to know I was just moments away from a whole new life?

I remember it still—that terrible night. The bathroom tiles making grout patterns in my knees as I hung onto the toilet bowl, throwing up from the sheer terror of my own life.

Alone.

Broke.

Unloved.

Lost.

Scared.

Oh, yes, and let's not forget, fat.

And as far from success as one could ever be.

Never had I imagined that my life road would lead me to this nasty motel room with its plastic ashtray, worn chenille bedspread, stained and smelly carpet.

Never would I have believed that the entire sum of my life could be stuffed into green garbage bags.

And never would I have believed that the size-eighteen-plus woman sitting on the bathroom floor with a fat lip, black eye, puffy ankles, smears of mascara on her face, and terror in her eyes would be me.

I was so scared I was numb.

I had run out of road.

I would have taken a whole bottle of pills, but the only ones I had packed were a tin of aspirins and a bottle of vitamin C and I couldn't remember which garbage bag I had thrown them into, and I didn't have the energy to look.

So I just huddled there afraid the night wouldn't end—afraid that it would. Now, I know that the next part of this story may sound a little strange—unbelievable, even. Miracles often do—

It began with the dawn. A soft sea light spread across the beach and drifted into that terrible room where I sat. It was getting lighter. I could see the stretch of sand and the foam-topped white-caps as they rolled into the shore. I could pick out clumps of dark-green seaweed and the pockmarks of clam shells. Far out I could see a small shrimp boat cross the horizon with its laddery crane.

I opened the sliding glass door of the motel room and stepped outside.

And that's when I heard it.

Not loud.

With no music.

Just the melody.

And the words.

An old hymn.

Remembered from my childhood.

"…I come to the garden alone.
While the dew is still on the roses.
And the voice I hear…."

The breeze blew away the next
words, and then, again the song picked up…

"…And He walks with me.
And He talks with me.
And He tells me I am his own…"

And that's when it happened. My
own personal miracle. I knew then and
there, on that early morning beach, that I
wasn't alone. That I wasn't unloved. That I
wasn't lost. He was right there, all along.

I turned back inside that motel room and took a good hard look at myself in the mirror. The smudged make-up. The stained blouse. The swollen and obese body. And then with His help, I looked beyond. I saw my future. I saw myself happy. Unafraid. Loved. Successful. Smiling. And in the mirror, that morning He even helped me see myself...SKINNY!

My life had changed, improved in minutes. That's how fast it happened to me. That's how fast it can happen to you. Starting right now!

Failure isn't falling down.
It's staying down.

Anon

What is important is to begin.

Hugh Prather

You may have to fight a battle more than
once, to win it.

Margaret Thatcher

If at first you don't succeed, you're running
about average.

M. H. Alderson

The Skinny Rules & You

If you can tell time, you can get skinny and stay skinny!

It's easy.
It's fast.
And it works.

All you have to do is follow my 7 Skinny Rules. That's it.

No dieting.
Nothing complicated.
Nothing stressful.
Just easy. Simple. Fun.
Nothing to measure.
Nothing to weigh.
Nothing to count.

You'll stop feeling guilty about food.
You'll start enjoying eating, again.
Your body will stop turning food into
        fat, and start turning it into
        energy.
You'll be able to go shopping
        in your favorite grocery store
        and buy skinny every day.

You'll be able to eat out, order in,
    enjoy parties, restaurants, and
    even those formerly terrifying
    buffets.
Every time you put a bite of food into
    your mouth, you'll be getting
    skinnier…more
    energized…happier…healthier
Your fridge will become your
    friend, not your enemy.
Your spouse and your kids can eat
    skinny right along with you,
    and never know it.

What a concept!

Again. If you can tell time, you can get skinny and stay skinny!

But there's even more. You're not going to be getting skinny alone. That's right. You've got me. And you've got my whole Skinny Team. Coaches, counselors, researchers—you've got a lot of friends here—all with one goal in mind, to help you get skinny and keep you skinny starting right now! So don't think you've got to do this alone. You've got friends.

That reminds me of a story I'd like to share with you.

It's about finding a friend when you most need one—it's a true story, because it happened to me. It's my favorite story about the power of a friend.

It was November, over twenty years ago and I was in New York City. I was looking for a job. I had two small babies to look after and the little money I had was quickly running out.

Day after drizzling day, I walked up and down those cold sidewalks, with no luck. By late afternoon of the fourth day, I realized that I had just enough money for another two days—if I was very careful.

It was getting dark, and a damp wind rushed through the trees of Central Park and chilled me through to the bone. I thought of a bowl of hot soup and turned a corner looking for a coffee shop, when instead, I found myself in front of the magnificent Plaza Hotel.

Something—maybe just the longing for warmth—pulled me inside. The lobby blazed with lights. Violins filled the air, competing gently with the sounds of laughter and the clink of crystal glasses and porcelain cups against fine china saucers. It was afternoon tea at the Plaza's famous Palm Court.

The maitre d' approached me and
without thinking I asked for a table for
one…a table for tea. A tea that would cost
me almost the rest of my precious money.
And so he seated me at a small table tucked
behind a giant palm, near the music.

And because I'm a talker, because I
was lonely, because I wanted so very badly
to connect with just one human being in that
cold, dark city, I started to chatter away.

I blurted out how I was looking for
work. That I had two babies at home I
needed to support. That this tea was costing
me the rest of my precious money—and a
bowl of soup in a coffee shop would have
been more sensible, but that I just wanted to

spend a few minutes in this enchanted room, where all the lights sparkled, all the people were beautiful, and the music filled my soul.

He didn't say a word, just left looking pretty stern, I thought. And I felt stupid for opening my heart and my mouth to a complete stranger.

But I eased my shoes off and pressed my toes into the warm, soft carpet. The music soared over me. For that moment I felt content. I felt as though I belonged. I closed my eyes.

When I opened them again, the maitre d' was standing in front of me. In one hand he held a bottle of French champagne and in the other a huge bowl of winter strawberries.

He placed both on the table in front of me, smiled and said, "Welcome to New York, compliments of the Plaza."

I looked at him and my eyes filled with tears of gratitude. And in that instant I knew I wasn't alone. I had a friend in that huge, cold city. I knew someone cared.

The next day I found a job. I made a home. I raised my two babies.

And every year I went back to the Plaza for tea. The lights would blaze. The music would soar. And I would slip out of my shoes and press my feet into the warm, soft carpet.

And every year, that same kind man who made me feel so very welcome on that lonely day served me a glass of French champagne and a bowl of strawberries.

And then he died.

Now, every year, in November I visit him. I bring a basket and together we share a bowl of winter strawberries and a glass of French champagne.

He was my friend and I was not alone.

Big Fat Lies—That Keep You Fat

I just get so mad, when I hear people repeating the same old stuff about their fat. Stuff they've been repeating for years.

So I decided to just make a list of what I call *big fat lies* that are at least partly responsible for keeping you fat and for stopping you from getting skinny fast and staying skinny.

Let's get rid of them all, right now.

Big Fat Lie

Eat Less—Weigh Less

How long is it going to take to figure out that starving yourself isn't going to get you any skinnier any faster—in fact, it's going to keep you fat, longer.

But still we keep right on trying these starvation diets. And every morning when we step on the scale, we still weigh exactly the same as we did the night before—or even more! That's when we ask ourselves for the thousandth time, "Why is it that the less I eat, the less I lose?"

Now I'm going to tell you.

Your body figures you are starving it and slows right down. The result? You get stuck. Your weight loss slows right down. You get frustrated. You cheat. You stay fat.

Big Fat Lie

Eating Fat Makes You Fat

You aren't getting fat from the fat you eat. In fact, you're probably eating less fat than ever. The *Department of Agriculture* reports that our total fat consumption has dropped by 17.5 percent. We're eating about 25 percent less fat than we ate thirty years ago and yet our obesity has increased by 25 percent.

What's going on? What's making us so fat?

Portions. We're getting fat from bigger portions. All those low fat, nonfat, reduced fat goodies are tempting us to eat more—that's one of the key reasons we're the fattest people on earth and getting fatter every day!

Big Fat Lie

Don't Eat After 6 PM

Good one.

Like your body knows that the donut you just scarfed down hit your tummy at 5:59 pm—and so it's not going to turn into fat.

But if you had swallowed it just one minute later—watch out—that same donut turns into an extra pound of fat and goes right to your middle!

The only clock-watching you need to be doing is coming right up and is designed to get you skinny—no matter when you eat!

Big Fat Lie

It's Not Me, It's My Fat Cells

Let's clear up the fat cell myth.

Fat cells aren't fat. In fact, fat cells are probably the skinniest cells in your whole body.

What makes them fat is that they are like balloons. Just a skim of wrapping around a space.

Keep them empty and they're flat, just like a balloon before you blow it up.

Fill them with fat, and they expand nice and round and puffy—just like a balloon filled with air.

The good news is that just like a balloon, you can empty your fat cells again and make them nice and flat, and skinny!

Big Fat Lie

All Fat Is The Same

Not exactly. In fact, there are two kinds of fat, but only one can actually help you get skinny fast.

We have what I call vanilla fat—whitish fat just under our skin, around our hips, bellies, thighs and buttocks.

We also have what I call strawberry fat—deeper fat, extending across our backs from arm pit to arm pit and wrapped around our vital organs.

This strawberry fat is critical in helping us get skinny. Once we start burning this deep strawberry fat, it burns hotter and uses more energy and consumes more fat calories and gets us skinny fast.

Big Fat Lie

I've Got A Slow Metabolism

This is my all time favorite big fat lie. The reality is, the fatter you are, the faster your metabolism works. The thinner you are the slower your metabolism.

Check it out for yourself with this simple formula to determine your Resting Metabolic Rate or RMR. This is the rate at which your body uses up calories while you sleep—this is your metabolism.

Your weight in pounds x 24 (hours in a day)
2.2 (kilograms)

Now give this same formula to your skinniest friend and see whose body uses up more calories—who has the faster RMR.

A good meal ought to begin with hunger
French proverb

One cannot think well, love well, sleep well,
if one has not dined well.
Virginia Woolf

If you have formed the habit of checking on
every new diet that comes along, you will
find that, mercifully, they all blur together,
leaving you with only one definite piece of
information: French fried potatoes are out.
Jean Kerr

Part Two

The Skinny Rules

Fat people die young.

Hippocrates

There is no wealth to compare with health of the body.

Ecclesiasticus 30:16

It is not the horse that draws the cart, but the oats.

Slavic Proverb

It is strange indeed that the more we learn about how to build health, the less healthy Americans become.

Adelle Davis

The Skinny Rules

Here they are.

The seven rules I have developed over years of helping Americans get skinny and stay skinny.

They are simple to follow.

They start working the very first day.

They keep working 24/7

They worked for me.

They will work for you.

Skinny Rule # 1

Set Your Clock To Skinny

If you can tell time, you can lose fat!

That's right. All you need to get started is your own watch, the most effective piece of fat-fighting equipment you can own. Timex or Rolex, it makes no difference. If it tells time, it can make you skinny.

Think of AM and PM as two new skinny food groups.

When your watch says AM, eat foods high in fiber. These foods help block new fat from being absorbed, clear out fatty arteries, and regulate the fat hormone, insulin.

When your watch says PM you'll eat foods high in protein. These thermic foods help burn off fat you've already got!

Skinny Rule # 2

Peel It Don't Pour It

Just making a simple switch from your usual morning orange juice to a whole orange can start you getting skinny even <u>before</u> breakfast.

Consider. Oranges are high in fiber—that white stuff that keeps the fresh juice in the orange—and fiber is a fat blocker.

Orange juice alone without the fiber, on the other hand, is often very high in sugar and sugar is a risk factor in obesity.

Just remember. Fiber can block fat. Sugar can make fat.

Skinny Rule # 3

Eat A Bedtime Snack

Would you like to wake up in the morning, skinnier than when you went to bed?

Sure. How? Simple.

Enjoy a high protein snack about an hour before going to bed.

The thermic or fat-burning properties of the protein raise your metabolic rate and can help your body burn off fat all night long.

So while you are sleeping, your own body's internal fat-fighting systems are hard at work helping you to get skinnier 24 hours a day, 7 days a week!

Skinny Rule # 4

Eat 7 Meals A Day

One meal. Two meals. Even three meals a day may be making you fat. By eating—7 meals a day—you can actually get skinny faster and stay skinny for good.

Here's what you do.

Eat often.

Eat fat blocking foods in the AM.

Eat fat burning foods in the PM.

The result?

You will not feel hungry or deprived.

Your metabolism will not slow down—instead, it will speed up, helping you to burn calories and lose fat quickly. So you can eat a greater amount of food. You can eat more often. And still lose fat, fast.

Skinny Rule # 5

Take Skinny Supplements

In a perfect world, you would be able to get everything you needed from your food.

But we don't live in a perfect world. We live in a world characterized by poor nutrition, lack of exercise, fatigue, and stress, all of which rob our bodies of the vital nutrients they need to be healthy.

That's why we need supplements. Supplements help your body do what it was designed to do. And these are my favorites:

Skinny supplements to fight fat.

Antioxidants to prevent disease.

Calcium to protect from osteoporosis.

Skinny Rule # 6

Think Skinny

Skinny begins in your mind.

Think yourself skinny…and your thoughts will become actions…and you'll be skinny.

See yourself skinny…and the picture you form in your mind's eye will be reflected in your mirror…and you'll be skinny.

Dream yourself skinny…and night after night your own subconscious will take up your skinny desire and your dream will come true…and you'll be skinny.

Skinny Rule # 7

Say A Skinny Prayer

There can never be total health for your body without health for your soul. It too, needs nourishment. So stop starving your soul. Feed it. Nurture it. Give it what it needs. And the whole of you—will be healthier and happier.

Whatever your faith. Whatever the words you choose. On your knees—or in your heart. In a cathedral—or in your own kitchen. Your soul is the key. Use it to unlock the body you want.

Simplify.

Henry David Thoreau

Part Three

Make The Skinny Rules Part Of Your Life

The future comes one day at a time.
Dean Acheson

The will to succeed is important, but what's even more important is the will to prepare.
Bobby Knight

If you want God to move a mountain, you'd better bring a shovel.

Anon

Have Dinner With Your Angel

Before you start making these simple rules a part of your new skinny life, I have one more story to share with you.

It's a story to savor before your first skinny dinner. Because it's then, in the evening, when we're most tired, stressed and hungry that all the good intentions of the day often disappear.

Enjoy.

It begins one spring evening.

But first, let me tell you about dinner. There's something about the dinner hour that cries out for company, for sharing the moments of the day that has just passed and for anticipating the evening that is to come. Dinner is to be shared, I always thought.

And so, if I didn't have a dinner companion—I just didn't have dinner.

Not a real dinner, anyway. I never set the table for myself—what was the point? I didn't cook for myself—again, what was the point?

More nights than I care to count found me standing at my open fridge prying

the lid off a pint of ice cream and spooning
it into my mouth right out of the container—
this was usually followed by a bag of
microwave popcorn and finally, the grand
finale—a heaping bowl of sugary cereal.

That was my usual dinner alone.

When I traveled, much the same
thing happened.

I never went out to a restaurant. I
was sure that everyone—the couples, the
families, the groups of friends—all averted
their eyes in pity when they saw me alone,
or with just a book for company.

So, when I traveled, I ate sitting up in
my hotel bed, propped up with pillows, the

room-service tray balanced on my lap, the television my only company.

But back to that spring evening.

It was late when I arrived in the small Southern town. I had been on planes all day and was starving. The only available hotel had no room service. The small grocery store was closed.

There was only one choice—eat out, alone.

It was a smallish restaurant. Warm. Crowded. Noisy. It was late enough that conversations flowing in that soft and gentle Southern cadence, quickened with wine and sweet iced tea, washed over the whole room and swirled around me as I stood alone at the entrance waiting to be seated.

I got my table, right in the middle of the floor—small, square, very conspicuous and set with two places.

There was nowhere to hide the fact that I was on my own. No one was coming to join me. No one was running late. It was as plain as it could be for everyone to see—I was eating my dinner alone.

A family sat at the table next to me with two small children. A boy, about nine or so, and a little girl, about five, looked at me as I tried to hide behind the menu.

The little boy piped up in that piercing voice that only small children have,

"Look Mommy, that lady has two plates, two cups, two saucers, two forks, two spoons—and she's eating all by herself."

Without missing a beat, his tiny sister glanced at me and then turned to him and said, "That lady isn't eating alone—she's eating with her angel."

And from that day to this, alone or with loved ones, I always set an extra place—because every night I have dinner with my angel.

How about you?

Your First Skinny Day

There are 7 meals in your skinny day.

1. Pre-Breakfast
2. Breakfast
3. Mid Morning Snack
4. Lunch
5. Afternoon Snack
6. Dinner
7. Bedtime Snack

AM

There are three meals in the AM.
Each meal is a high fiber meal.
Each meal blocks fat.

Meal 1	Pre-breakfast
Meal 2	Breakfast
Meal 3	Mid morning snack

PM

There are three meals in the PM.
Each meal is a high protein meal.
Each meal burns fat.

Meal 5	Afternoon Snack
Meal 6	Dinner
Meal 7	Bedtime Snack

Lunch

To block or to burn—that is the question!

AM or PM?

What time is it?

Lunch is the meal with an identity crisis. Is it an AM meal or a PM meal? Is it the time to keep blocking fat or to start burning fat?

The answer to this question is up to you.

Lunch time is the one meal of the day we just don't have much control over. We sometimes have to rely on the office microwave to heat up some leftovers from last night's dinner. Or, we may only have time to grab a sandwich at the fast food joint around the corner.

No problem! As long as you eat either an AM <u>OR</u> a PM meal, you're still on your way to Skinny!

At lunchtime, block fat <u>OR</u> burn fat…the choice is yours!

Your Skinny Plan

Meal 1   Pre-Breakfast - Fat Blocker
1 orange or 1 apple or 1 pear

Meal 2   Breakfast - Fat Blocker
Oatmeal with brown sugar, or
Waffles with syrup, or
Pancakes with syrup, or
Toast or bagels or muffins, with jelly

Meal 3   Morning Snack - Fat Blocker
Fruit salad, or
Oatmeal cookies, or
Popcorn, or
Raisins

Meal 4   Lunch - Fat Blocker
Salad and/or veggies
Veggie sandwich, or
Soup with crackers, or
Beans with toast, or
Veggie chili with a bagel, or
Meatless Mexican or Chinese food

OR

Meal 4   Lunch - Fat Burner
Salad and/or veggies
Eggs or
Chicken, tuna, or egg salad, or
Grilled hamburger patties, or
Fish, chicken, pork, lamb, or beef

Meal 5   Afternoon Snack - Fat Burner
Cheese or Yogurt, or
Meat or fish, or
Eggs, or
Peanut butter

Meal 6   Dinner - Fat Burner
Salad and/or Veggies
Meat or Fish, or
Cheese, or Eggs

Meal 7   Bedtime Snack - Fat Burner
Peanut butter, or
Deli meats, or eggs and/or cheese

Best AM Fat Blocking Foods

Breads	Cereals
Waffles	Oatmeal cookies
Pancakes	Raisins
Apples	Oranges
Pears	Kiwi Fruit
Berries	Tortillas
Popcorn	Fig cookies
Brown rice	Potatoes
Corn	Peas
Beans	Lentils
Grapefruit	Pasta
Dried fruit	Carb sports bars

Best PM Fat Burning Foods

Lean red meat   Pork
Chicken   Turkey
Lamb   Fish
Tofu   Cheese
Yogurt   Skim milk
Eggs   Peanut butter
Protein bars

Supplements

Here are my personal picks.

Fat Fighting Supplements
Chromium
L'Carnitine
Garcinia Cambogia (Citrimax®)
Chitosan
Citrus Aurantium

Antioxidants & Vitamins
Vitamin C
Vitamin E
The B Vitamins

Minerals
Calcium
Iron

Sleep Supplements
Chamomile
Kava Kava
Melatonin

That's Your Whole Skinny Solution™

See how easy it is to get skinny and stay
skinny 24/7 from the first day to forever.
Follow my *Skinny Rules.*

Just set your clock to skinny.
Eat AM fat blockers.
Switch to PM fat burners.
Take your skinny supplements.
And develop an attitude…a skinny attitude!

A big skinny thank you from me to all of
you—oh yes, and my angel says "thanks"
too!

Get The Skinny

To shop in my Skinny Store™ or become a member of my Skinny Club™. Log on or call toll free. It's fast. It's friendly.

www.skinny.com

1-888-7-SKINNY